BARTO

Fats

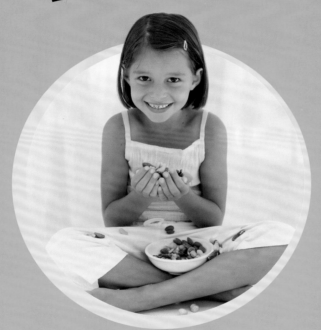

George Ivanoff

Smart Apple Media
P.O. Box 3263
Mankato, MN, 56002

First published in 2011 by
MACMILLAN EDUCATION AUSTRALIA PTY LTD
15–19 Claremont St, South Yarra, Australia 3141

Visit our web site at www.macmillan.com.au or go directly to www.macmillanlibrary.com.au

Associated companies and representatives throughout the world.

Copyright Text © George Ivanoff 2011

Library of Congress Cataloging-in-Publication Data has been applied for.

Publisher: Carmel Heron
Commissioning Editor: Niki Horin
Managing Editor: Vanessa Lanaway
Editor: Emma Short
Proofreader: Georgina Garner
Designer: Kerri Wilson
Page layout: Cath Pirret Design
Photo researcher: Sarah Johnson (management: Debbie Gallagher)
Illustrator: Leigh Hedstrom, Flee Illustration
Production Controller: Vanessa Johnson

Manufactured in China by Macmillan Production (Asia) Ltd.
Kwun Tong, Kowloon, Hong Kong
Supplier Code: CP December 2010

Acknowledgments

The author and the publisher are grateful to the following for permission to reproduce copyright material:

Front cover photograph: Girl eating nuts, Photolibrary/Stockbyte

Photographs courtesy of: Dreamstime, 25 (middle), /Angelsimon, 29 (bottom), /Bellafotosolo, 12, /Bradcalkins, 28, /Casaalmare, 29 (top), /Cybernesco, 7 (middle), /Dusanzidar, 24, /Elenathewise, 25 (right), /Ginosphotos, 22 (right), /Icefront, 7 (bottom left), /Iofoto, 18, /Kivig, 9 (fish), /Miradrozdowski, 9 (nuts), /Monika3stepsahead, 8, /Monkey Business Images, 20, /Og-vision, 11, 14 (olive oil), /Olgapshenichnaya, 14 (almonds), /Photosoup, 27 (right), /Sangiorzboy, 15 (fish), /Tysmith, 27 (left), /Ukrphoto, 3, 7 (bottom), / Valentyn75, 7 (bottom right), /Viktorfischer, 9 (butter, cream), /Valentyn75, 25 (left); Getty Images/Purestock, 21; iStockphoto/Daniel Loiselle, 22 (left), /Catherine Yeulet, 30; Photolibrary/Banana Stock, 13, /Graham Kirk, 26; Pixmac/a4stockphotos, 6 (top), / Alexander Silaev, 7 (top); Shutterstock/Elena Elisseeva, 15 (flaxseed oil), /greenland, 19, /marco mayer, 10, /Morgan Lane Photography, 6 (middle), /Monkey Business Images, 5, 17, /paulaphoto, 4.

While every care has been taken to trace and acknowledge copyright, the publisher tenders their apologies for any accidental infringement where copyright has proved untraceable. They would be pleased to come to a suitable arrangement with the rightful owner in each case

Contents

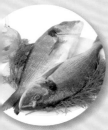

When a word is printed in **bold**, you can look up its meaning in the Glossary on page 31.

What's in My Food?

Your food is made up of **nutrients**. Nutrients help your body work, grow, and stay alive.

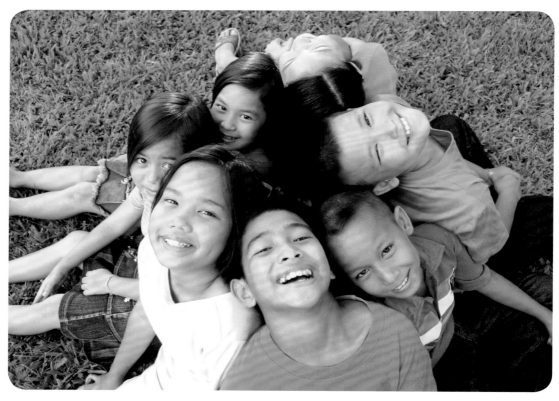

Nutrients give you **energy** so you can be active.

Different types of food contain different types of nutrients. A **balanced diet** includes foods with the right amount of nutrients for your body.

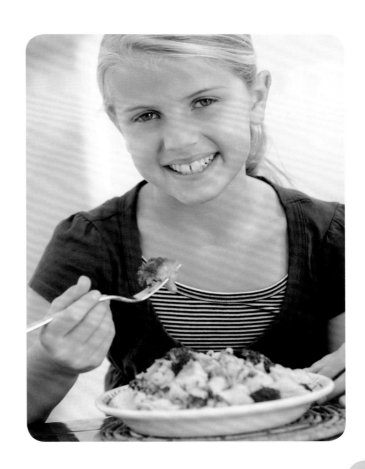

A balanced diet helps keep your body healthy.

What Nutrients Are in My Food?

There are many different types of nutrients in your food. They include proteins, carbohydrates, fats, fiber, minerals, and vitamins.

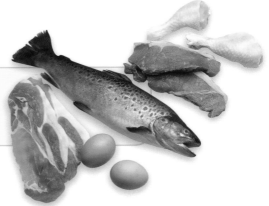

Protein in meat, poultry, eggs, and fish helps your body grow and heal.

Carbohydrates in bread and pasta give your body energy.

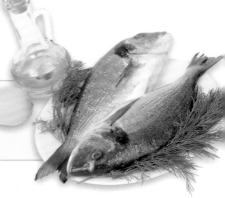

Fats in fish and olive oil give your body energy and help it stay healthy.

Fiber in bread and vegetables helps your body **digest** food.

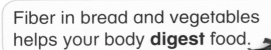

Vitamins in fruit and vegetables help your body work well.

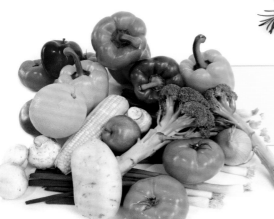

Minerals in milk and meat help your body grow and stay healthy.

Fats

Fats are nutrients that are found in many foods. Your body needs fats to stay healthy.

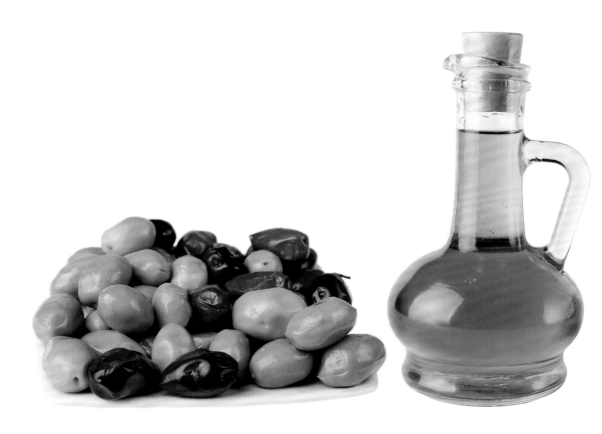

Olives and olive oil contain healthy fats.

Some fats are good for your body. Other fats are not as good for your body. You should eat less of these types of fats.

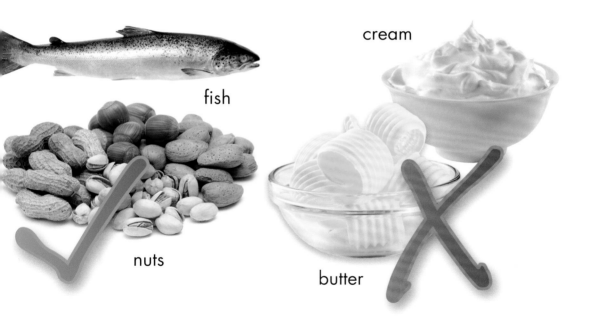

cream

fish

nuts

butter

These foods have good fats.

These foods have fats that are not as good for you.

What Are Fats?

Fats are made up of a liquid called glycerol and smaller parts called fatty acids. Fats are **macronutrients**. Your body needs a lot of macronutrients to stay healthy. Protein and carbohydrates are also macronutrients.

Fats, as well as protein and carbohydrates, can be found in a meal of bread, chicken, and salad with dressing.

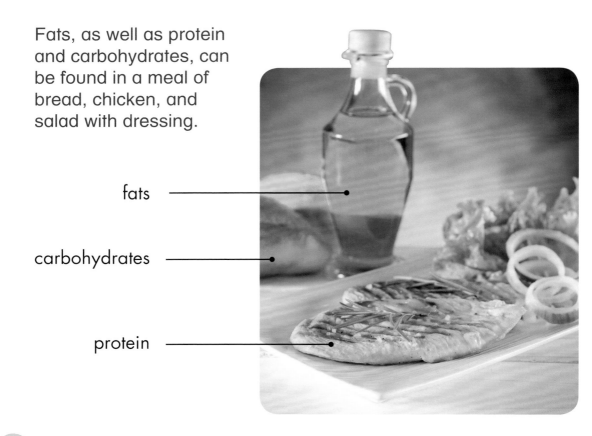

fats

carbohydrates

protein

Different foods have different types of fats. There are three main types of fats: saturated fats, unsaturated fats and trans fats. Some foods contain more than one type.

The fats in olive oil are made up of saturated and unsaturated fats.

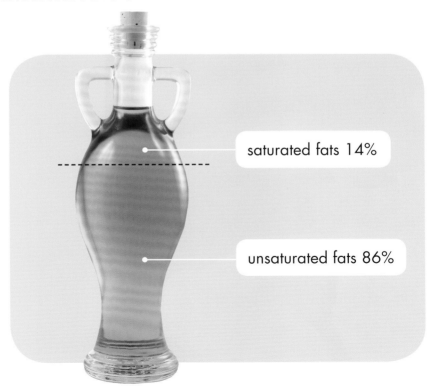

saturated fats 14%

unsaturated fats 86%

Saturated Fats

Saturated fats contain fatty acids that build up **cholesterol** in your body. You should not eat too many saturated fats.

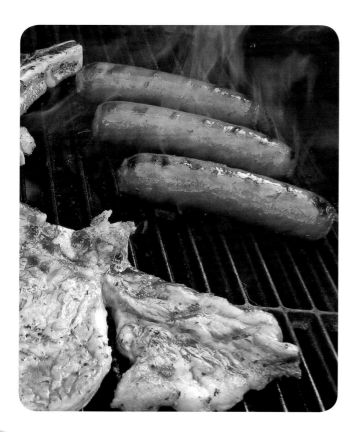

Meat has a lot of saturated fats.

Trans Fats

Trans fats are made from **processed** vegetable oils. They increase your cholesterol and the risk of heart **disease**. You should not eat too many trans fats.

Many fast foods contain trans fats.

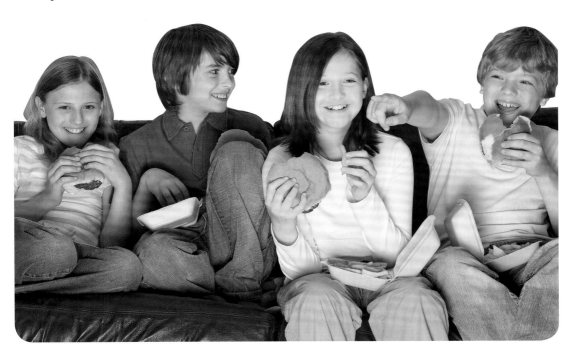

Unsaturated Fats

Unsaturated fats contain fatty acids, but they don't build up cholesterol in your body. They are the most healthy type of fats.

These foods contain unsaturated fats that help keep your heart healthy.

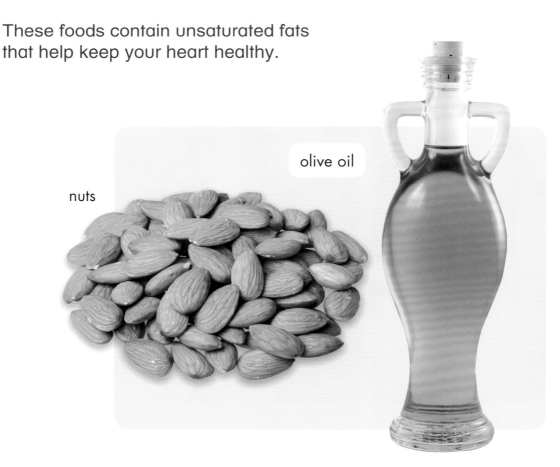

olive oil

nuts

There are two types of unsaturated fats: polyunsaturated and monounsaturated fats. Some polyunsaturated fats contain a fatty acid called omega 3. Omega 3 is very good for you.

Oily fish, flaxseed, and flaxseed oil contain omega 3.

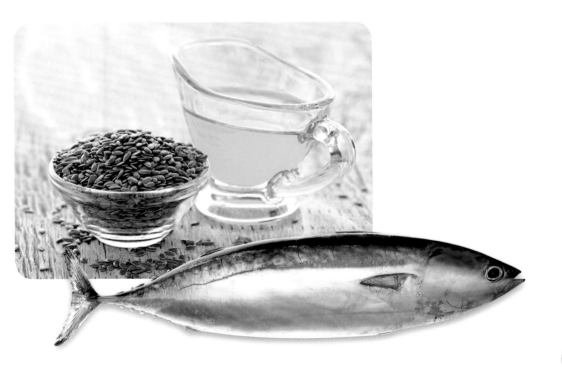

How Does My Body Get Fats?

Your body **absorbs** fat when you digest food. When food breaks down in your stomach, the fats break down into fatty acids. The fatty acids enter your blood.

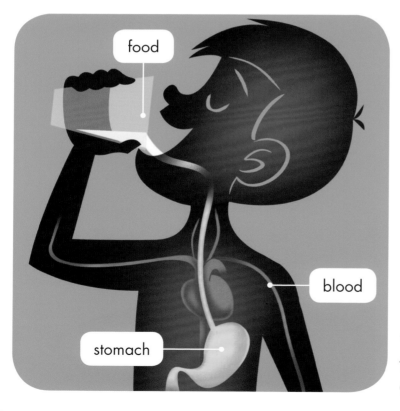

food

blood

stomach

Your blood carries fatty acids all around your body.

The fats your body does not need are stored in your **fatty tissue**. They can be used later when they are needed. If more fat is stored than your body can use, you can become overweight. Your body uses fats in three ways:

1. Fats give you **energy**.

2. Fats help your body absorb vitamins.

3. Fats help you grow and keep your body healthy.

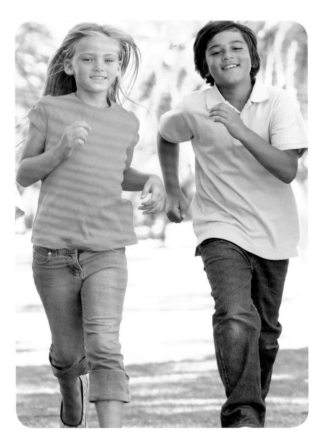

What Do Fats Do?

Fats give you energy and power your brain. They also help your body absorb the vitamins it needs to stay healthy.

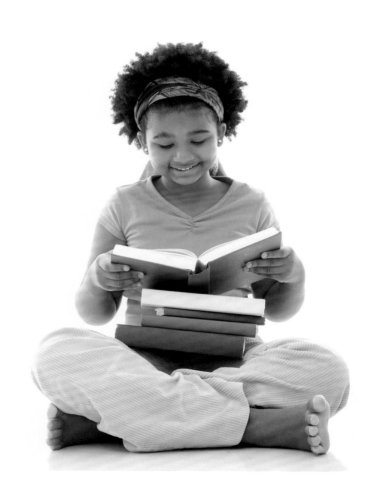

Fats help your body absorb vitamin A, which gives you good eyesight and healthy skin.

Fats Power My Body

Some fats give your body energy. They help it move, work, and stay active.

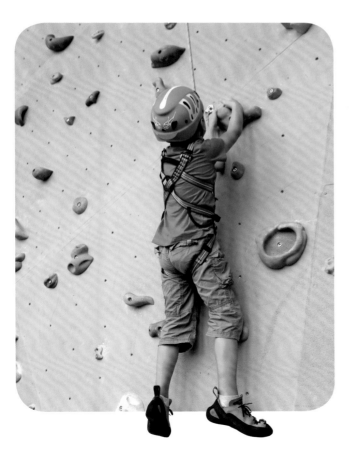

When you haven't eaten for a while, your body uses its stored fats for energy.

Fats Keep My Brain Healthy

Fats help build the brain and **nervous system.** They keep both healthy.

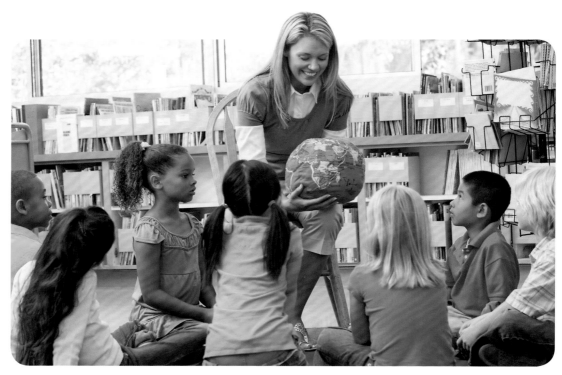

Children need more fats than adults because their brains and nervous systems are still growing.

Fats Help My Body Absorb Vitamins

Fats help your body absorb the vitamins that it needs. Your body needs fats to absorb vitamins A, D, E, and K.

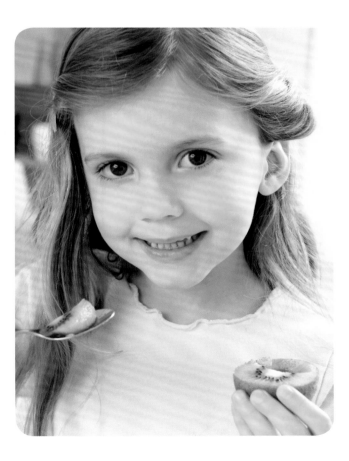

Kiwi fruit contains vitamins A, C, and E, and omega 3.

Which Foods Contain Fats?

Lots of foods contain fats. Different foods have different types of fats, and your body uses them in different ways. You need to eat foods with fats every day.

All these foods contain fats, but some types of fats are healthier than others.

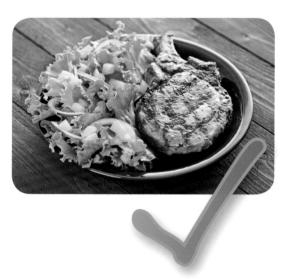

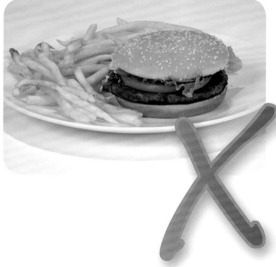

Foods with fats are part of a balanced diet. Other foods also have nutrients that your body needs, such as vitamins and minerals. You need to eat these foods, too.

A balanced diet includes many different kinds of foods, as well as water.

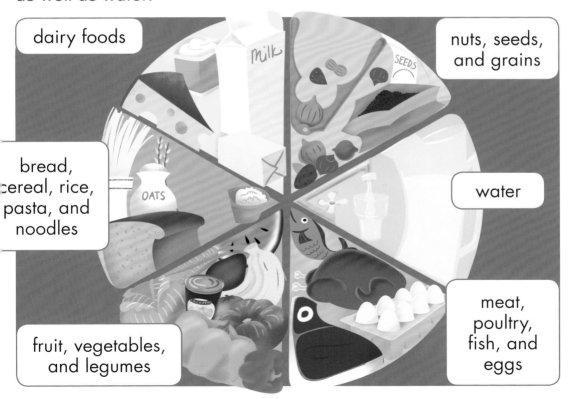

dairy foods

nuts, seeds, and grains

bread, cereal, rice, pasta, and noodles

water

fruit, vegetables, and legumes

meat, poultry, fish, and eggs

Fats Are in Oily Fish

Fish contains polyunsaturated fats and omega-3 fatty acids. Omega 3 is very good for your body and keeps your heart healthy.

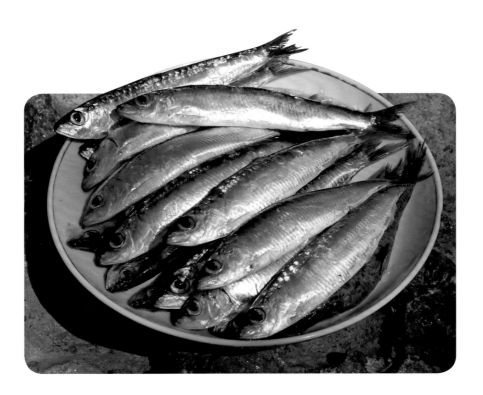

Oily fish such as mackerel, salmon, tuna, and sardines contain omega 3.

Fats Are in Oils

Vegetable oils that have not been processed contain unsaturated fats. Olive oil has a lot of monounsaturated fats.

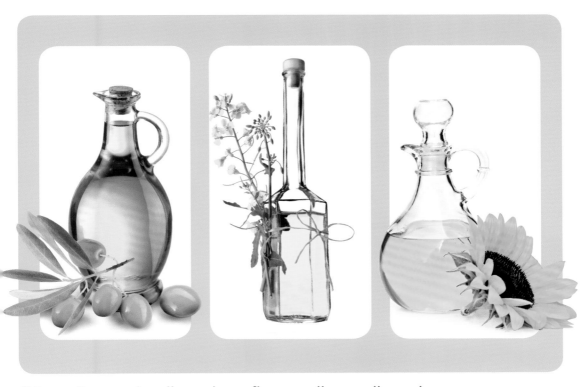

Olive oil, canola oil, and sunflower oil are all made from plants.

Fats Are in Meat, Poultry, and Dairy Foods

Meat and poultry contain saturated fats. Your body needs only a small amount of saturated fats. You should not eat too much of them.

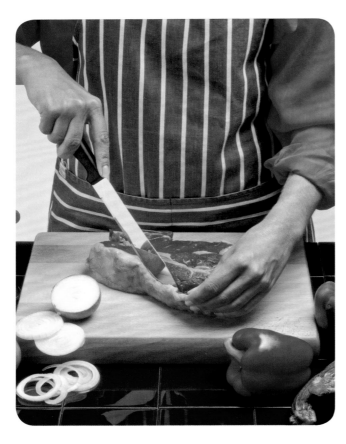

Cut off the fatty parts of meat and poultry before cooking.

Dairy foods are made from milk. Dairy foods contain saturated fats, but some also have nutrients, such as minerals and protein.

Milk has less saturated fats than cream, so it is more healthy.

milk

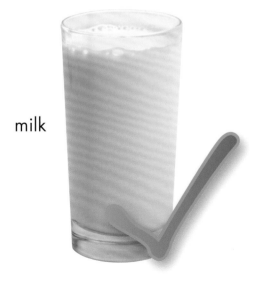

cream

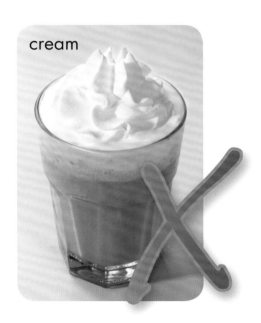

Fats Are in Fruits and Vegetables

Some types of vegetables, called legumes, contain fats. Soybeans and chickpeas are legumes. They have unsaturated fats. Avocados and olives also have unsaturated fats.

chickpeas

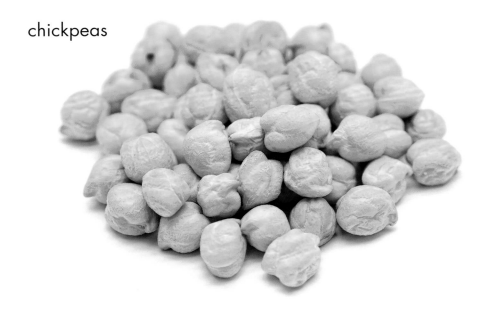

Chickpeas are legumes, which contain unsaturated fats.

Fats Are in Nuts and Seeds

Some nuts, such as coconuts, have saturated fats. Others, such as hazelnuts, have healthier unsaturated fats. Sesame seeds, safflower seeds, sunflower seeds, and flaxseeds have unsaturated fats, too.

Different types of nuts have different amounts of saturated and unsaturated fats.

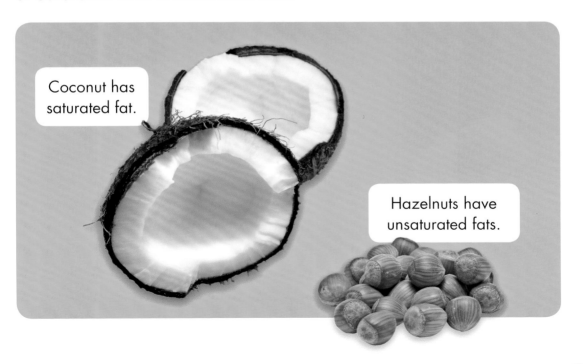

Coconut has saturated fat.

Hazelnuts have unsaturated fats.

What Happens if I Don't Eat Fats?

If you don't eat fats, your body won't have energy.
Your brain and nervous system won't work well.
Your body won't be able to absorb vitamins that
keep it healthy.

If you don't eat any fats, you won't have
enough energy to be active.

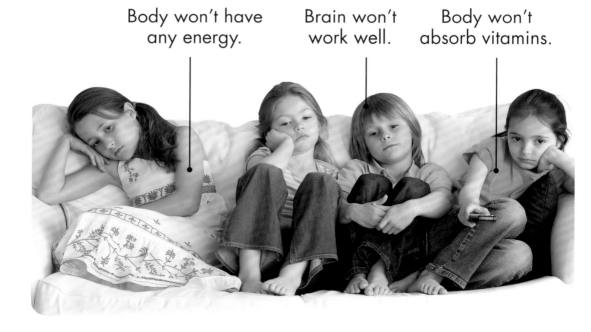

Body won't have
any energy.

Brain won't
work well.

Body won't
absorb vitamins.

Glossary

absorbs	takes in
balanced diet	a healthy selection of food that you eat
cholesterol	a substance in your blood and brain that can build up and cause health problems
digest	to break down food in your body
disease	an illness or sickness
energy	the ability to be active
fatty tissue	parts of your body where fat is stored
macronutrients	nutrients that your body needs a lot of
nervous system	the system that sends messages between your brain and body
nutrients	the healthy parts of food that you need to live
processed	changed in some way

Index